INFLAMMATION

The Silent Killer

Holly Fourchalk, PhD., DNM®, RHT, HT

DISCLAIMER

Every effort has been made by the author to ensure that the information in this book is as accurate as possible. However, it is by no means a complete or exhaustive examination of all information.

The author knows what worked for her and what has worked for others but no two people are the same and so the author cannot and does not render judgment or advice regarding a particular individual.

Further, because our bodies are unique any two individuals may experience different results from the same therapy.

The author believes in both prevention and the superiority of a natural non-invasive approach over drugs and surgery.

The information collected within comes from a variety of researchers and sources from around the world. This information has been accumulated in the Western healing arts over the past thirty years.

Research has shown that one of the top three leading causes of death in North America occurs because of the physician/pharmaceutical component of the scenario.

Perhaps the real leading cause of death and disability is a result of the lack of awareness of natural therapies. These therapies are well known to prevent and treat many common degenerative, inflammatory and oxidative diseases.

The author loves to research and loves to teach. This book is another attempt to increase awareness about health and the many options we have to bring the body back into a healthy balance.

Ever-increasing numbers of people are aware of healing foods and herbs, supplements and modalities but there are still far too many who are not. The fact that our physicians are part of this latter group makes healing even more challenging yet we are now seeing more and more laboratories around the world and more universities in and outside of the U.S. studying herbs, nutrition and various healing modalities with phenomenal success.

The unfortunate fact is, those who can profit from sickness and disease promote ignorance and the results are devastating.

use of any of the suggestions or information contained in the book but offer this material as information that the public has a right to hear and utilize at its own discretion.

To my Parents

For all their support and encouragement
My Dad for his ever-listening ear
My mother for her open mind

INDEX

ONE

Introduction to the
Inflammation-Immune-Gut systems

Did you know that your inflammatory system, immune system and gut system are intimately interconnected?

Did you know that your body is constantly provoking and eliminating inflammation?

Did you know that it is estimated that about 98% of doctor visits are actually due to functional medicine and most of that has to do with the inflammatory response?

Did you know that the inflammatory response is an important part of your immune system?

Did you know that the microbes in your gut can and do alter your DNA, your chromosomes, your genes?

Did you know that the inflammatory response is an important part of your body's complex biological response to a wide variety of situations?

Did you know that simply lying down on a bed and breathing will break the smallest of the arteries (arterioles) and cause an inflammatory reaction?

Did you know that inflammation is a complex biological response to harmful stimuli, like pathogens, damaged tissues or cells?

Did you know that if your immune system were not functioning well, your inflammatory response mechanism would go awry?

Did you know that about 90% of your immune system is in your gut?

Did you know that the immune system is the cause of allergies?

Now, how did we get from inflammation to the immune system to the gut? Well, let's take a look at how they are all interconnected, how they can go astray, *and* how we can resolve the problem.

TWO

The Inflammatory Response

Most of us have had an experience of inflammation. Whether as a child falling off a bike or out of a tree, or as an adult slipping, falling or some other kind of an accident, we have all experienced a "booboo".

We are usually familiar with the classical signs of inflammation:

- Pain
- Heat
- Redness
- Swelling

But did you know that the inflammatory response is the body's way of protecting you, getting rid of a harmful stimuli, and initiating a healing process?

The initial inflammatory response is called an acute response. Hopefully, it is short lived and resolved effectively. Unfortunately, too many times it is not and for a wide variety of reasons.

If the inflammatory response process is not effectively resolved, we end up with chronic, ongoing, unresolved inflammation. Whether this is a chronic inflammation or a subclinical inflammation it can cause long-term damage. There are several reasons this may occur.

It is this prolonged chronic inflammation that is usually the concern in alternative medicine.

Several dysfunctions in the body are inflammatory in nature. These include:

- Asthma
- Bursitis
- Celiac disease
- Crohn's disease
- Diverticulitis
- Gastritis
- Gingivitis
- Laryngitis
- Otitis
- Polymyalgia rheumatic
- Rheumatoid arthritis
- Tendonitis

Other diseases may not be inflammatory in nature, but rather have an inflammatory component, for instance:

- Alzheimer's
- Atherosclerosis
- Cancer
- Diabetes mellitus
- Obesity

Chronic inflammation can be subtle, or subclinical, i.e., you can have it for years and not even be aware of it. For instance, you may have a bone break that never fully healed, or an infection that never fully healed. You may have metal or other chemical toxicities that keep accumulating and the body cannot eliminate them. That's when the inflammation becomes a "subclinical inflammation" that is never resolved but continues to cause a host of other problems.

You may have chronic inflammation that you are well aware of but experiencing a difficult time resolving, such as, rheumatoid arthritis, atherosclerosis, hay fever or even cancer. All have an inflammatory component. MDs will usually give you prescriptions, many of which are addictive, to attempt to manage the symptoms but nothing to resolve the underlying issues.

Whether you are aware of the inflammation or not, unresolved inflammation can be dangerous. So let's look at the inflammatory response a little more carefully.

With this next part, you want to understand the general concepts. You are *not* going to be tested on these terms. You do want an overall understanding of the different types of roles each component plays in the system.

When inflammation is initially stimulated, a huge number of substances and systems like to get involved and we don't want to leave anything out. Let's start with the blood – your vascular system.

Your *vascular system* is comprised of all the blood vessels in your body.

- Oxygenated blood leaves the heart through the aorta and is carried through the arteries throughout your body.
- Veins carry the toxins and CO_2 back to the heart and lungs, entering the heart through the vena cavae.
- The average adult has about 5 – 6 quarts (4.7 – 5.7 liters) of blood in his or her body.
- The blood consists of:
  - Red blood cells carry oxygen (through the body) and CO_2 (out of the body)
  - White blood cells (immune cells)
  - Plasma
  - Platelets

The *blood or vascular* system is very involved in the inflammatory response mechanism. The blood carries a large number of compounds identified as the "biological cascade of molecular and cellular signals" that both trigger and resolve the inflammatory response."

At the site of trauma, injury or infection, blood cells will release molecular "signals" that provoke a number of changes in the area:

1) Vasodilation – expansion of the arteries allowing for:
   - Increased blood flow
   - Vascular permeability – meaning the artery walls loosen up to allow various compounds to pass through and help the process
   - Exudate: proteins and antibodies permeate through the blood vessels into the affected area

Then the *immune system* gets involved:

1. Various signalling molecules (cytokines) call different compounds to the area:
   - Neutrophils (a type of white blood cell/leukocytes) are involved in the initial stage of inflammation and focus on infection.
   - Some neutrophils release other cytokines which keep the process going:
     i. Interleukin (IL) -1
     ii. Interleukin (IL) – 6
     iii. TNF (tumor necrosis factor)
     iv. INF-gamma (gamma interferon)

Then the *liver* gets involved:

2. Some pro inflammatory cytokines provoke the liver to produce (synthesize) various "acute phase reactant proteins" which may provoke:
   - Fever
   - C-reactive protein
   - Increase or decrease coagulation factor depending on what is required

Back to the *Immune System* again:

3. Some neutrophils directly attack pathogens:
   - Ingest them (phagocytes)
   - Release pathogen toxins (peptides and proteins)
   - Generate traps and act as free radicals on the invading infection)
4. And then we have the backup team of other leukocytes (including granulocytes, monocytes and lymphocytes) that are called to the area.

These molecules are all involved in the inflammatory response. But *chronic* inflammation can occur if:

1. Viral or bacterial infection is not resolved
   a. Pathogens can travel in the blood and get into joints.

b. Pathogens can get into joints from wounds, injections and surgery.

c. Pathogens can also last for years.

2. These pathogens can develop into an auto-immune disorder whereby the immune system gets confused and starts attacking compounds that are part of the system.

3. Persistent aggravation of the situation whereby the healing repeatedly gets interrupted, i.e. someone going back to exercise or work too quickly can also cause problems.

4. When we don't have the nutrients/ molecules required to solve the problem.

   a. Most immune cells for growth, maintenance and response require glutathione. If there is insufficient glutathione then all these molecules fail to respond effectively.

   b. We don't have sufficient proteins in the body to make the immune cells.

   c. The liver is compromised (fatty liver disorders, cirrhosis, inflammation, etc.) whereby it cannot support the Immune system.

   d. The adrenals are compromised and cannot regulate the immune system.

e. The gut is compromised and we do not absorb the nutrients we need to support the immune system.
f. We have metal and other toxicities that prevent the immune system from functioning (note the majority of the immune system is in your gut).

So, even with just a simple overview of the inflammatory response mechanism, we can see how various different aspects of the body join together in a distinct, integrative dance to help resolve the problem at hand.

THREE

Biomarkers for Inflammation

There are many different tests to determine the level of inflammation in the body. These are called "biomarkers of inflammation".

1. Acute-phase reactant proteins: CRP, SAA, vWF antigen, fibrinogen.
2. White Cell count (different immune cells).
3. ESR (erythrocyte sedimentation rate) which is the rate at which red blood cells sediment or break down in one hour – a non specific test of inflammation.
4. Albumin is the most abundant blood plasma protein. If ESR and white blood cells are high and albumin is low, we have inflammation. Albumin helps repair damaged tissues, transports various molecules like fatty acids and cortisol, and stops the blood fluids from leaking out of your blood vessels.
5. Cytokines are signalling molecules, i.e. IL-1 beta, IL-6, IL-18, TNF-alpha, increase in order to tell the rest of the system what the local area needs in order to heal the inflammation.
6. Adhesion molecules, E-selectin, P-selectin, ICAM-1, VCAM-2, increase so that molecules

come to the area to support the adhesion required to mend the wound.

Abbreviations:

CRP (C-reactive protein) *a blood protein that increases with inflammation.*

ESR – Erythrocyte Sedimentation Rate – *the rate at which blood cells sediment in a one hour period and indicative of inflammation.*

ICAM-1 – Intercellular Adhesion Molecule – 1 aka CD54 – *ICAM refers to the gene that expresses the cell surface glycoprotein, which occurs on immune cells and blood vessel cells.*

IL – Interleukin – *a group of cytokines or signalling proteins, many of which are produced by leukocytes.*

SAA – Serum Amyloid A-protein – *a group of apolipoproteins (fat-proteins) associated with HDL (good cholesterol) produced by the liver and seen in acute phase inflammation.*

VCAM-1 – Vascular Cell Adhesion Molecule 1, a.k.a. Vascular Cell Adhesion Protein 1 – *a group of proteins that connect or bind cells together.*

vWF – von Willebrand Factor – *a group of blood glycoprotein (sugar-proteins) that tend to be deficient or defective in von Willebrand disease, thrombosis,*

Heyde's syndrome and increase with cardiovascular, blood, and connective tissue diseases.

FOUR

Nutrient Factors in Inflammation

There are many dietary concerns that may play a part in inflammatory conditions. For instance, most of us have heard of the need for Omega 3 fatty acids, which are anti-inflammatory. There are many other factors as well. This chapter is going to take you through a simple process of understanding the different types of:

- Fats
- Fatty acids
- Omega 3s

Fats are a group of compounds derived from fatty acids and glycerol called triglycerides. Any given fat molecule will have specific properties concerning the fatty acids that make it up. The type of fatty acid will determine the impact it has on the body.

A basic triglyceride pictorial representation looks like this:

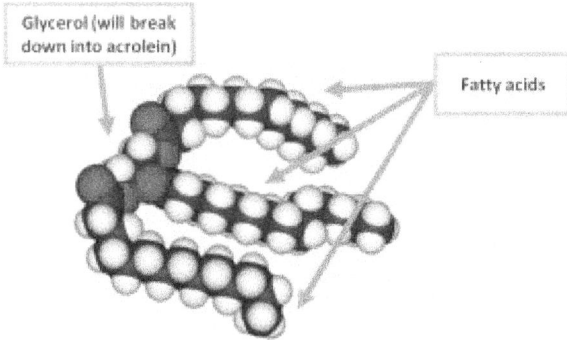

Glycerol (will break down into acrolein)

Fatty acids

Whereas a chemistry diagram looks like this:

Triglyceride

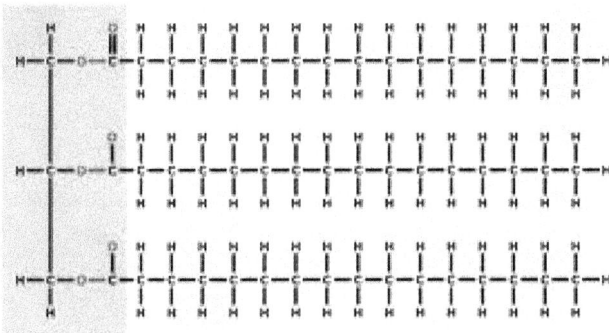

It is amazing how neither looks anything like this:

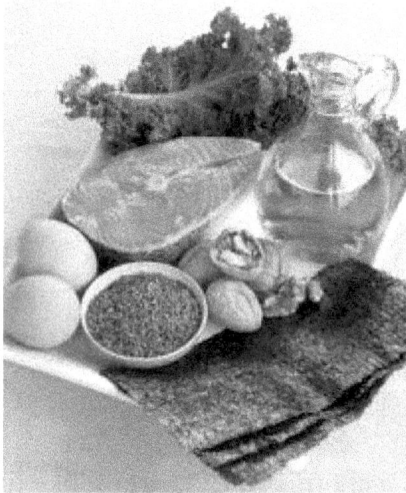

Or conversely like this:

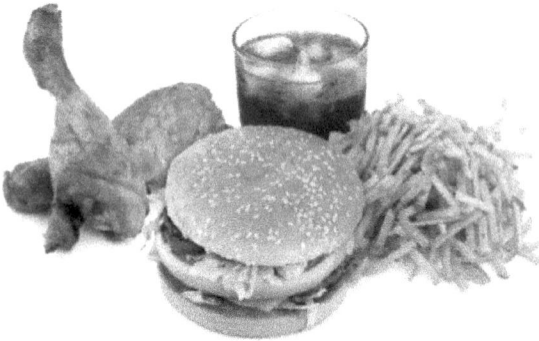

So what are the differences, if they are all fats?

Saturated fats differ in the carbon to hydrogen ratio. If each carbon molecule is saturated with a hydrogen molecule then it is a saturated fat. These occur in:

- Cream
- Cheese
- Butter
- Indian Ghee
- Fatty meats

If the fat contains double bonds within the carbon chain then we have an unsaturated fatty acid. These includes:

- Monounsaturated fats:
  - Almond oil
  - Grape seed oil
  - Olive oil
  - Sesame oil
  - Sunflower oil
  - Cashews
- Polyunsaturated fats:
  - Walnuts
  - Sunflower seeds
  - Sesame seeds
  - Peanut butter
  - Salmon
- Trans fats (typically the result of processing, although there are some in nature, such as

when hydrogens are on the opposite side of the carbon):
- o Baked goods
- o Fast foods
- o Fried foods
- o Snack foods
- Cis fats (placement of the hydrogens on the carbons – hydrogens on the same side of the double bond):
  - o Most of the naturally occurring unsaturated fats
- Omega fatty acids:
  - o Omega 3s (anti-inflammatory):
    - Chia seed oil
    - Flax seeds and oil
    - Grains
    - Green leafy vegetables
    - Hemp seed oil
    - Mustard seeds
    - Pumpkin seeds
  - o Omega 6 (inflammatory):
    - Chia seed oil
    - Grape seed oil
    - Hempseed oil
    - Safflower oil
    - Sunflower oil
  - o Omega 9 (reduces hardening of the arteries, improves immune function, lowers cholesterol):

- Avocados
- Almonds
- Cashews
- Chia seeds and oil
- Olives and oil
- Pecans

Note the many foods have a combination of a variety of different Omegas. Nature rarely operates in isolation but rather is wonderfully integrative, which in and of itself should teach us something. Our diets, right down to our fats, should be a broad mixture.

- Polyunsaturated fatty acids have more than one double bond, thus the term "poly".
- Unsaturated fats can turn into saturated fats through a process called hydrogenation and thus we have products like margarine.

So how does all this impact on us? Well, saturated and unsaturated fats differ in their energy, the melting point, and their impact. Unsaturated fats provide less energy but saturated fats pack themselves close together.

What do healthy fats do in the body?

- Provide transport vehicles for vitamins and other nutrients.

- Insulate neurons so that they work faster and more effectively.
- Provide structure for hair and nails and skin.
- Help regulate body temperature.
- Provide structure for the membrane of every cell in the body.
- Provide the basis for many hormones.
- Provide energy (the glycerol component is used as fuel).
- Protection against toxins.

While this is not an exhaustive list it provides a range of functions for which we require fats.

Now let's look at a specific type of fat: Omega 3.

Omega 3

What exactly is an Omega 3 fatty acid? The 3 in Omega 3, like the 6 in Omega 6, or the 9 in Omega 9, simply indicate where the first double bond occurs in the carbon chain.

However, there is much more to it than that.

For instance, when researchers first did cardio experiments with fats, they used Omega 6, not realizing that Omega 3 fatty acids are anti-inflammatory and Omega 6 fatty acids are inflammatory. Of course, the results they got reflected this but no one understood what they were actually researching. The knowledge came after all the hoopla that fats were so bad for us!

We now know that there are unsaturated and polyunsaturated Omega 3 fatty acids which act as anti-inflammatories. (Note: The saturated fats and trans fats have the opposite impact on the body – pro-inflammatory!) The Omega 3s are considered essential, as the body cannot produce them. Yet, they are vital to our metabolic processes. There are different types of Omega 3s, so let's go further.

Some food sources of Omega 3 fatty acids are:

- Fish, algae, and squid oil
- Flax, Hemp and Chia oils and seeds
- Hazel, Pecan and Persian walnuts
- Cocoa (whole and not processed)
- Eggs (if fed on greens and insects versus corn and soybeans)
- Meat (if grass fed/grazed versus grains)

But, there are different types of Omega 3s that the body requires:

Dark green leafy vegetables +

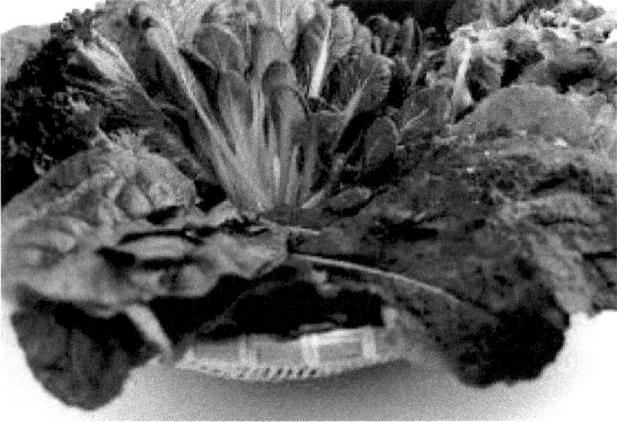

Flax seed, Hemp seed, Chia seeds +

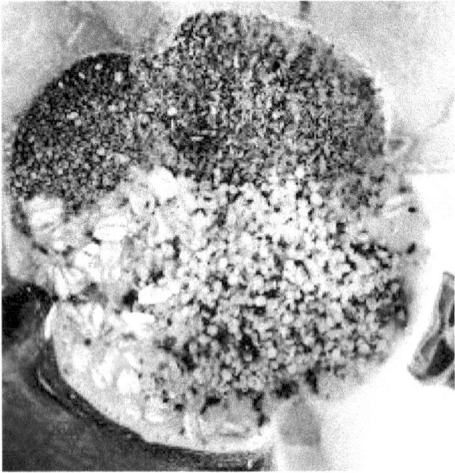

Good healthy oil: olive oil, walnut oil, and coconut oil.

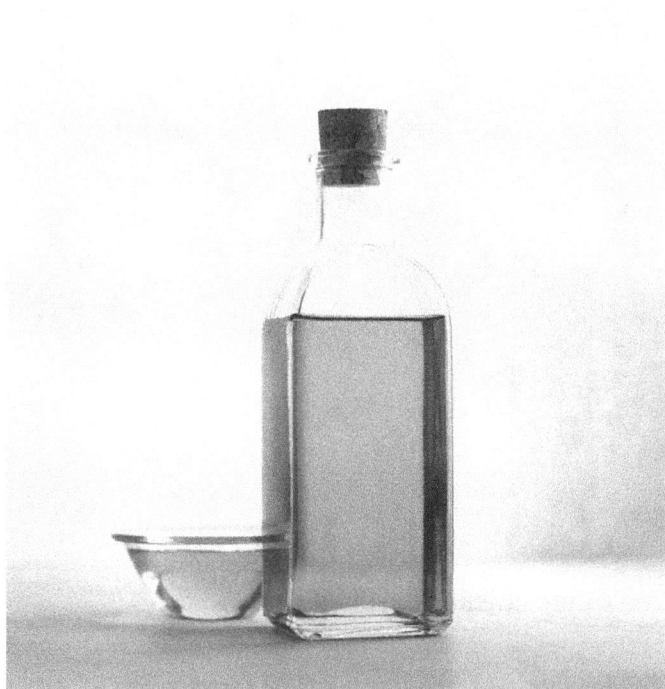

All provide ALA or Alpha Linoleic Acid. The body then converts the ALA into different intermediate compounds. These compounds are then converted into EPAs (EicosoPentaenoic Acid), which the body converts back and forth with DHAs (Docosahexaenoic Acid) as required.

We get both EPAs and DHAs from: Cold water fish (salmon, cod, krill, mackerel, tuna) +

Various kinds of seaweed +

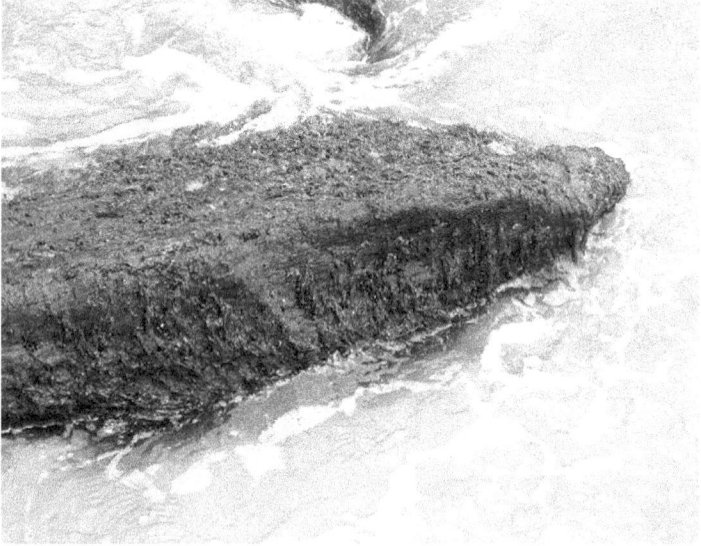

Free range chickens and eggs +

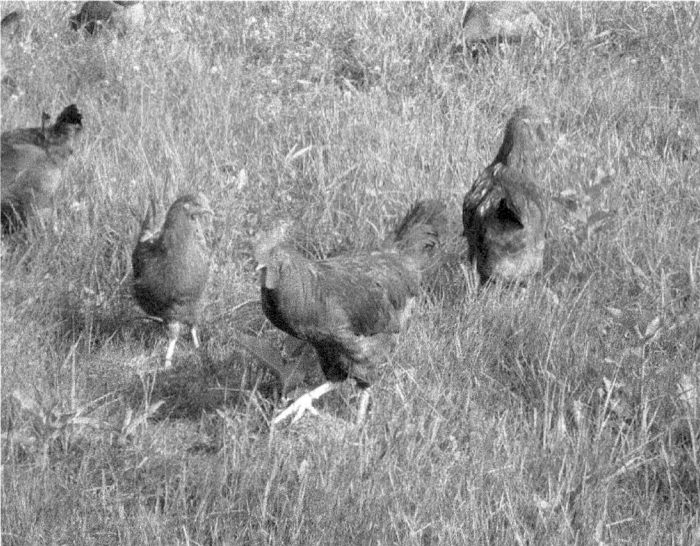

Grass fed cattle +

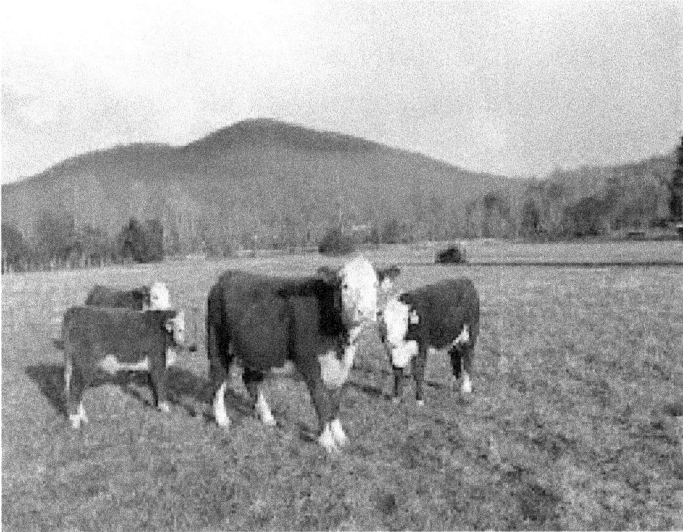

Xocai™ Omega chocolate squares=2oo mgs of DHA.
So the resulting diagram might look like this:
ALA -> x,y and z -> EPA ⇔ DHA

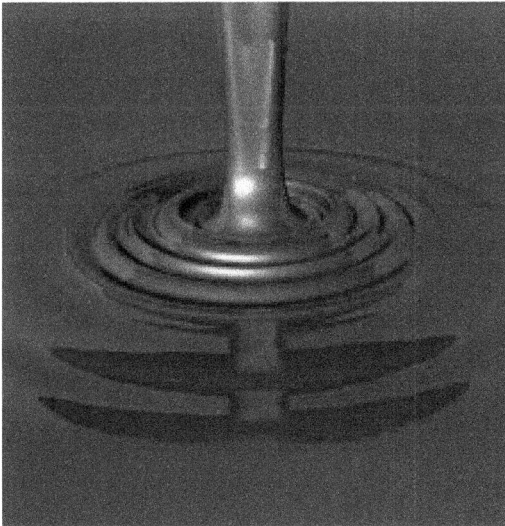

Overall, studies report that a Mediterranean diet is high in:

- Good olive oils (Note: most of the olive oils in North America have lost their Omega 3 fatty acids for which they are acclaimed.)
- Beans
- Fish
- Fresh, organic fruits and vegetables
- Nuts and seeds (preferably raw and unsalted versus roasted)
- Whole grains

Many conditions have shown a significant improvement with the use of Omega 3 fatty acids:

- ADHD
- Autism spectrum disorders
- Bipolar disorders
- Cardio disorders: hypertension, varicose veins, etc.
- Dementias
- Depression (significantly low levels of DHA)
- Development conditions
- Rheumatoid arthritis

There is a lot of controversy over the degree to which we can convert ALA to EPAs and DHAs. Therefore, to utilize a broad spectrum diet wherein you get all the fatty acids is the most effective.

What do ALA, DHA, EPA and DPA do in the body?

ALA: Alpha linoleic acid is found in the highest concentrations in plant food oils. The following chart is taken from:
http://en.wikipedia.org/wiki/Alpha-linolenic_acid

Common name	Alternate name	Linnaean name	% ALA[†]	ref.
Chia	chia sage	*Salvia hispanica*	64%	[9]
Kiwifruit seeds	Chinese gooseberry	*Actinidia chinensis*	62%	[9]
Perilla	shiso	*Perilla frutescens*	58%	[9]
Flax	linseed	*Linum usatissimum*	55%	[9]
Lingonberry	cowberry	*Vaccinium vitis-idaea*	49%	[9]
Camelina	camelina	*Camelina sativa*	35-45%	
Purslane	portulaca	*Portulaca oleracea*	35%	[9]
Sea buckthorn	seaberry	*Hippophae rhamnoides L.*	32%	[10]
Hemp	cannabis	*Cannabis sativa*	20%	[9]
Rapeseed	canola	*Brassica napus*	10%	[2]
Soybean	soya	*Glycine max*	8%	[2]
			[†]average value	

The primary function of ALA is to provide the precursor for both EPA and DHA. But it also accumulates in various body parts, i.e. adipose fat and skin, and it is recognized for its function in the neural and cardio systems. Evidence suggests that increased levels are correlated with lower levels of cardiovascular disease and cancer.

Note: There is a similar fatty acid called linoleic acid and is found in greater concentrations in the fatty tissues (perhaps because the ALA gets converted to DHA and EPAs).

DHA can be found in maternal milk and fish oil.

The most abundant Omega 3 fatty acid is found in the brain (40%) and the retina of the eyes (60%). To be more specific 50% of the neural membrane is composed of DHA.

DHA is also involved in the transport of *choline, glycine* and *taurine*.

Choline, often grouped with the B complex vitamins, which are important in:

- Prevention of fatty liver disorders (alcoholic and non-alcoholic)
- Structural integrity
- The signalling between cells
- Important for production of *acetylcholine*
    o A neurotransmitter in the brain

- To slow heart rate
- A precursor for the SAMe pathways (produced and consumed by the liver and involved in more than 4 metabolic reactions)
- At neuromuscular junctions

Glycine: The smallest of 20 amino acids (basics of proteins).
- Thus important for making proteins
- Provides a base unit for the purines (two of the four nucleotides that make up the DNA)
- Acts as an inhibitory neurotransmitter

Taurine: Structurally considered an amino acid but not technically.
- A major component of the bile produced by the liver and stored in the gallbladder, and released into the colon to digest fats.
- Plays a role in: Anti-oxidation, cardiac function, membrane stabilization, and regulating calcium signalling, osmoregulation, skeletal muscle function, retina.

In addition, DHA is involved in potassium channels, synaptic vesicles, cell death, especially in the brain (apoptosis), sperm head formation (which holds the enzymes that penetrate through the egg).

In general fatty acids are shown to:

- Help strengthen cell membrane integrity

- Help repair cellular and tissue damage
- Help optimize neurological transmission and brain function
- Help improve heart and circulatory function
- Help produce supple, moist skin
- Aid retinal function and response to light
- Aids lung function

It is important to recognize how interactive the system is. We started out talking about various types of fats and ended up talking about various types of amino acids and their various roles from the brain to the liver to muscles and the circulatory system.

Unfortunately, allopathic medicine has become so reductionistic that the program appears to forget how interactive the whole system is.

Thus, in addition to predominantly managing symptoms rather than eliminating the underlying causes, they also only usually only look at one protocol rather than recognizing that if you are finally in a place where you are recognizing the symptoms, the body has done a lot of compromising along the way.

Again, in most alternative healing modalities, practitioners recognize the basic six stages of illness. They work at distinguishing what stage the illness has progressed to and what needs to be done to restore harmony and balance to the whole body –

versus simply eliminating your perception of symptoms.

In today's society, too many people want immediate gratification, akin to the pleasure principal (no perception of symptoms) and they don't want to take responsibility for their health. They would rather "do what they please" and then let the health practitioner or the MD "take care of the consequences".

As a result, we have ended up as one of the unhealthiest civilizations in history. People think we are actually living longer but if we eliminate the dramatic change in mortality during the first year of life, statistics show that we are living one week longer than previous generations lived.

So much for all that scientific research! The statistics for longevity are tremendously misleading as well. When we eliminate the infant mortality statistics then it appears that we really do live longer but when we include from the moment of birth (regardless of whether you are premature or not) then we don't live longer. For a simple overview on the different types of statistical analysis utilized in determining longevity, go to:

http://www.nationalrighttolifenews.org/NewsOnli ne/June-July2011/AmericanHealthCare.html

As the old saying goes: "Figures don't lie until statisticians start to figure".

Or conversely: "Statistics are like bikinis. What they reveal is suggestive, but what they conceal is vital."
Aaron Levenstein

One statistical quote that I particularly like is: "Statistics - A subject which most statisticians find difficult but in which nearly all physicians are expert."

Fibre

Now fibre is an immensely important factor in the health of the gut and just like fats, for a wide number of reasons.

To begin with, there are two major types of fibre:

- **Soluble,** which regulates the blood glucose uptake in your liver, dissolves in water, can be fermented in the gut and cause gas, and can be prebiotic.
- **Insoluble,** which helps regulate the transit of your bowel movements, does not dissolve in water, provides prebiotics, and metabolically ferments in the colon.
- **Most fibre foods contain both soluble and non-soluble fibres but are categorized according to which is more predominant.**

Let's focus on the role of the insoluble fibre. These fibres can change the characteristics of the contents in the intestines. They can alter how various nutrients are absorbed. Fibres, like lignins, can also alter the metabolic rate.

One of the major benefits of fibre is the production of necessary compounds as a by-product of the fermentation process.

Fibre itself provides compounds like:

Beta – glycan: Beta-glycans are a type of polysaccharides that are known for their anti-tumour capacity, ability to modulate the immune system, and regulation of blood cholesterol. They are found in various mushrooms (reishi, shiitake, and maitake), baker's yeast, oats and barley.

Chitins: A derivative of glucose; helps to improve the balance of gut microbes, thus improving metabolic processes and thereby aids in reducing weight. They are found in the walls of fungi and the skeletons of crabs, lobsters, and shrimp.

Dextrins: By-product of starch or glycogen (through hydrolysis), or produced from starch using enzymes (amylases). Increases good digestive bacteria, reduces cholesterol and other fats, reduces blood sugar levels, regulates the insulin response, helps to fight colon diseases, involved in the detox process.

Food sources include: Starch from corn, sweet potatoes, and tapioca subjected to a hydrolysis process (using water to break chemical bonds).

Inulin: A type of polysaccharides (fructooligo-saccharide) produced in many plants. They belong to a group called fructans, usually found in the roots of plants and used as a mean of storing energy. In humans, helps the growth of gut bacteria. Can be found in agave, banana, burdock, dandelion, garlic, onion, and wild yam.

Oligosaccharides: Compounds of 2-10 simple sugars, part of glycoproteins (sugar/protein) and glycolipids (sugar/fat) compounds, provide food for the intestinal flora – some types stimulate gut flora and other types suppress them. They are found in asparagus, Jerusalem artichoke, burdock, leeks, onions.

Pectins: A type of soluble fibre *and* a type of heteropolysaccride (meaning more than one type of monosaccride in the structure) found in the walls of plants; binds to cholesterol in the intestinal tract and slows the absorption of glucose by trapping carbohydrates. Found in carrots, peas, cucumbers, celery, tomatoes, and legumes.

Waxes: Plants grown in warmer areas, produce a wax to control evaporation and dehydration. Found in Brazilian palm, sugarcane, jojoba, honeycomb, leaves and stems of major grain crops.

If you have eaten too much fibre, you may experience gassy bloating, but the result of too little fibre is constipation.

Although it is important to realize that there are many other causes for constipation as well.

FIVE

Inflammation and Gut Microbiota

Alternative healing modalities will focus a lot on the gut and inflammation. Western medicine is finally catching up. Ayurvedic medicine had a good understanding of this over 3000 years ago—and well documented.

If the gut is on fire, every system in the body is going to be affected. Intestinal inflammation/fire can be the cause of:

- Allergies
- Alzheimer's
- Arthritis
- Autism
- Autoimmune diseases
- Behaviour disorders
- Cancer
- Depression
- Diabetes
- Heart disease
- Mental illnesses

Why? How? Well, it is somewhat more complicated than previously thought.

1. The bacteria/microbes in our gut share their genes with us.

2. A microbiome is the total number of microbes (with their genetic components) – their genes outnumber ours.
    a. We have 10^{12} number of cells in the body.
    b. There are 10^{13} number of microbes in the body.
    c. That means there are ten times more of them then us. Or, in other words, they outnumber our cells 10 to 1.
    d. Their combined gene load is about 10 million. Humans have about 25,000 genes so we are definitely out numbered, again.
    e. These microbes have an impact on the way your body:
        i. Metabolizes foods
            1. Sugars
            2. Carbohydrates
        ii. Detoxifies chemicals
        iii. Metabolizes hormones
        iv. Obtains and uses nutrients
        v. Controls some of your DNA.

The following is a chart from http://en.wikipedia.org/wiki/File:Skin_Microbiome20169-300.jpg that identifies the major categories of microbes in the body:

Actinobacteria
  Corynebacterineae
  Propionibacterineae
  Micrococcineae
  Other Actinobacteria
Bacteroidetes
Cyanobacteria
Firmicutes
  Other Firmicutes
  Staphylococcaceae
Proteobacteria
Divisions
contributing < 1%
Unclassified

(Gb) Glabella
(Al) Alar crease
(Ea) External auditory canal
(Na) Nare
(Mb) Manubrium
(Ax) Axillary vault
(Ac) Antecubital fossa
(Vf) Volar forearm
(Id) Interdigital web space
(Hp) Hypothenar palm
(Ic) Inguinal crease
(Um) Umbilicus
(Tw) Toe web space

Retroauricular crease (Ra)
Occiput (Oc)
Back (Ba)
Buttock (Bt)
Gluteal crease (Gc)
Popliteal fossa (Pc)
Plantar heel (Ph)

Front   Back

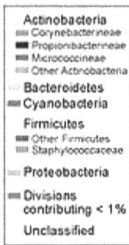

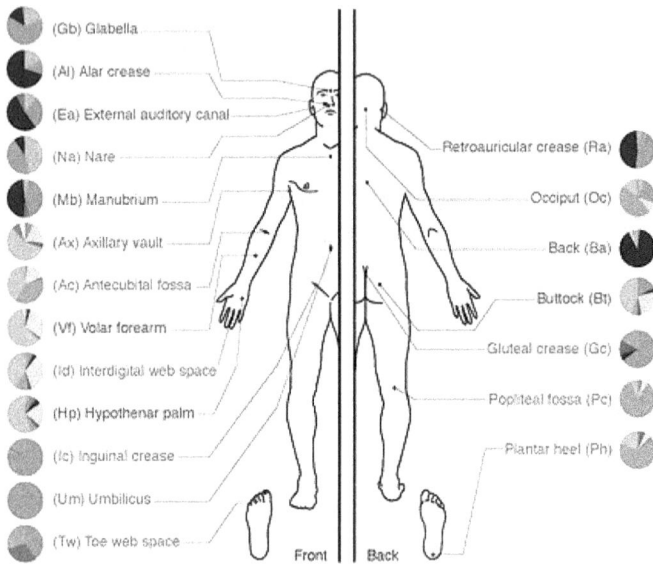

In short, these microbes can determine both gut inflammation and immunity. Wow! No wonder so many different healing modalities focused on the gut.

So we know that the immune system is supposed to stand to attention when bacteria, parasites, viruses, toxins, etc. get out of control. The first part of the immune reaction usually includes an inflammatory response.

But...if the problem isn't readily resolved, if the toxins keep coming, if the diet continues to be deficient, if the processed, microwaved, pasteurized foods keep coming then the inflammation never gets resolved and becomes *chronic*.

When we further create dysfunction in the gut:

- By taking Anti-biotics
- By taking antacids
- Drinking acidic water carrying toxins
- Overworking the adrenals that help regulate the immune system
- Overworking the liver that supports the gut with enzymes and bile.

We are literally killing ourselves.

Chronic inflammation is a killer! It is passive. It is subtle. And it can be deadly.

SIX

Microbes and the Immune System

Your immune system has different components.

Innate immunity, non-specific immune system:

- First line of defense
- Defense mechanism for responding to pathogens, such as viruses, bacteria, mould, fungus, etc.
- Involves bringing immune cells to the problem area to identify and respond and eliminate the pathogen/germ
- Provoking the initiation of the complement cascade system that identifies the pathogen
- Involves the different types of white blood cells to remove the pathogen
- Provokes the adaptive immune system, if necessary
- Provides a barrier to the chemical or pathogen in order to protect the body
- Includes the inflammatory response mechanism which is considered a stereotyped response versus a learned adaptive response (adaptive immune system)

Adaptive immunity, specific immune system:

- This system is different than the generalized innate immune system because it:
    - Involves highly specific cells
    - Systemic cells/processes that eliminate pathogens
    - Has a memory of pathogens that have invaded before
        - Therefore will respond stronger each time the pathogen presents itself
    - Is a system that learns and is therefore considered adaptive

So already you have learned that the inflammatory response is part of the innate immune system.

Immune system: **A variety of immune cells.**

- Dendritic cells
- Histiocytes
- Kupffer cells
- Macrophages
- Mastocytes

Then we have the inflammatory mediators (typically responsible for the redness and heat because they cause the arteries to dilate, also known as vasodilation.

- Cytokines: various types of small proteins that communicate or "signal" cells although they are neither hormones or growth factors
- Chemokines: a particular group of cytokines signaling proteins. There are four types, but either operate to maintain homeostasis or inflammation
- Histamine: released from Mast cells in response to an allergic reaction causing an inflammatory response
- Leukocyte eicosanoids: a specific type of signaling molecule that control inflammatory and/or immune responses
- Lysosome: hold onto toxins in a cell
- Macrophage cytokines called TNF (tumor necrosis factor) and ILs (Interleukins)
- Nitric oxide (a gas released from macrophages, endothelia cells and neurons)
- Prostaglandins from mast cells: a localized hormone aka autocrine or paracrine that regulates insulation and muscle relaxation

Fish oil **decreases inflammatory cytokine secretion.**

- *Turmeric (curcumin)* and *Bovine colostrum* (transfer factor) inhibit C-reactive protein, Il-6, Il-1, PBMCs.[1]

SEVEN

Microbiota and the Gut

We have already identified that there are many different types of bacteria throughout the gut. What we now know is that the gut microbiota provides a number of functions from:

Protective functions:

- o The outer membrane layer of the intestine is made up of mucins or glycoproteins, proteins made from the microbes.

Immune functions:

- o Develop and regulate the host's defences.
- o Contribute to the regulation of the immune system.
- o Impacts the interaction between the outer layer of the gut (epithelium) and the lymph tissue (part of the immune system).
- o The epithelial layer of the gut provides a physical barrier to our bodies and regulates what we absorb and what we need to eliminate.
- o The membrane (outer layer) of the gut consists of the mucosal epithelial membrane, which secretes mucus that aids in the passage of the food.

Metabolic functions:

- o The microbes in the gut affect the host's metabolism.
- o Provides additional/required enzymes.
- o Contributes to the regulation of gene expression (those genes involved in the utilization of carbohydrates and lipids, the utilization of non-digestible carbohydrates and sugar compounds, regulation of bile acids, cholesterol reduction, synthesis of vitamins (K and B vitamins), drug bioconversion, etc.[1]

We need to feed these microbes and it appears that many of them feed on complex polysaccharides (various plant sugars).

Fermentation of these polysaccharides provides short-chain fatty acids and various gases that support cell growth and differentiation.

Let's look at what different levels of different bacteria are associated with:

1. There are different population densities between thin and obese people. Obese people have a significantly reduced variety of bacteria plus an increased level of enzymes, with increased efficiency of calorie harvest.

2. Type 1 diabetes is associated with:
   a. Dysfunctional intestinal bacteria
   b. Leaky gut syndrome

    c. Difference in immune responsively

3. Autoimmune children (including Type 1 Diabetes) show the following:
    a. Unstable gut microbiome
    b. Significantly reduced levels of biodiversity
    c. Firmicutes replaced by Bacteroidetes

4. A proposal was put forward to classify people by enterotype, meaning based on the composition of the gut microbiome.

Now for the really "wow" information…research is now showing that our gut is not in control of our microbes but rather many of the microbes control the immune system! For instance, different microbes control an important part of the immune system cell called the *T helper 17 cells*.

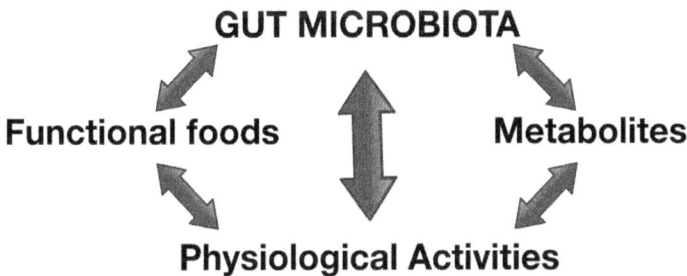

GUT MICROBIOTA

Functional foods   **Metabolites**

Physiological Activities

In alternative medicine, we are forever looking at the originating factors. Whether we look at Ayurvedic, Traditional Chinese Medicine (TCM), ancient African, and ancient Egyptian healing modalities, all looked to the gut. As a side note –

they all claim to be the oldest. Hippocrates, the father of western medicine, claimed, "food is your medicine and medicine is your food". He also claimed, "cure sometimes, treat often, comfort always". In Appendix 1, you will find a number of quotes about healing. It is always a wonder how modern medicine forgot the basics claimed by the father of western medicine.

In today's alternative healing modalities (or traditional healing) we still look to the gut.

EIGHT

Metal Toxicity and the Gut

We keep hearing of toxicity but are you aware of all the different types of toxicities? Some metals we require:

- Chromium – needed for enzymes
- Cobalt – needed for Vitamin B12; co-enzymes
- Copper – co-factor in enzymes
- Iron – hemoglobin, myoglobin
- Selenium – enzymes, insulin receptors
- Zinc – enzymes, immune systems

However, there are various other heavy metals that are toxic to the body. This chapter will explore the different types of metal toxicities and the impact that they have on your gut and your body.

One of the reasons heavy metals become toxic and impair your body's capacity to function is that they replace nutrients in the enzyme binding sites. In order for any compound, molecule, etc. to break down or build up into something we need, enzymes are required. We have over 10,000 enzymes and co-enzymes in our body. So you can imagine the problems that can arise when an enzyme is blocked from functioning.

When heavy metal toxins block enzymes or receptors for enzymes, they either over-stimulate the receptor *or* prevent the receptor from being stimulated. Either way these toxins alter thousands of enzymes in the body.

These heavy metal toxins may also cause problems by simply accumulating and depositing in various sites, tissues, organs, etc. where they cause irritation, inflammation and dysfunction, and again, alter normal functioning.

Another problem that may occur is when we are deficient in one type of necessary mineral, i.e. zinc, the body will then use cadmium, lead, or mercury instead of zinc and cause all kinds of other issues. For instance, when cadmium fits into zinc binding sites of important enzymes like RNA transferase, carboxypeptidase, alcohol dehydrogenase, and others, we are in for trouble.

Another example is arsenic, which binds to red blood cells and globulins (a required type of blood protein).

While the heavy metal is helping us to continue function in the short term, problems begin to evolve over time.

Now, an additional issue is the compounding effect of these heavy metals. For example, it has been shown that, not only are mercury and lead extremely toxic to the cells and to the brain, but when combined their impact is significantly worse. One study gave sufficient mercury to kill 1% of the rats – and it did. They then gave sufficient lead to kill 1% of the rats – and it did. But when combined, this dose killed 100% of the rats![1]

Other heavy metals do the same, i.e. cadmium and arsenic, or other toxic chemicals like PCBs, pesticides, and tobacco smoke. How about when the mercury, thimerosal, found in vaccines, was combined with the aluminum also found in vaccines?[2]

The challenge is that our soils are becoming more and more depleted of the nutrients we need and thus, the plants that feed our bodies are more and more deficient, so our bodies are more and more willing to uptake the harmful metals to supposedly compensate – in the short term.

Considering that our diet is full of these heavy metals, never mind synthetic pharmaceutical drugs, vaccinations, etc. the first processing of them occurs in the gastrointestinal tract, which is where a lot of the inflammation begins.

In addition, these metals DO NOT biodegrade AND they accumulate, thus causing more and more problems.

First here is a generalized list of common signs and symptoms of heavy metal toxicity:

- Alcohol intolerance
- Allergies (both food and environmental)
- Anxious and irritable
- Brain fog

- Cannot lose weight
- Chronic unexplained pain
- Coated tongue
- Cold hands and feet
- Dark circles under the eyes
- Depression
- Digestive problems
- Extreme fatigue
- Frequent colds and flus
- Headaches
- High levels of toxic metals in your blood, urine and tissues
- Insomnia
- Intolerance to medications and vitamins
- Loss of memory and forgetfulness
- Low body temperature
- Metallic taste in your mouth
- Muscle and joint pain
- Muscle tics or twitches
- Muscle tremors
- Night sweats
- Parasites
- Prone to moods swings
- Sensitive teeth
- Sensitive to smells
- Skin problems
- Small black spots on your gums
- Sore or receding gums
- Tingling in the extremities
- Unsteady gait
- Vitamin and mineral deficiencies

What this list shows us is how many different systems in the body can be affected by metal toxicities.

Now let's look at the individual metal toxins. The World Health Organization identifies ten chemicals that are "of major health concern" and these include:

- Air pollution
- *Arsenic*
- Asbestos
- Benzene
- *Cadmium*
- Dioxin and dioxin like substances
- Fluoride
- *Lead*
- *Mercury*
- Highly hazardous pesticides[3]

The following is a brief on the heavy metals in this list, where we find them, and the symptoms they cause:

Aluminum – Is often associated with memory loss and the various dementias. Aluminum effects our:

- Gut: Reduces intestinal activity and may cause colic.
- Nervous system: Blocks the action potential in a neuron which prevents the secretion of neurotransmitters; it may also prevent the re-uptake of various neurotransmitters, and it inhibits various neural enzymes.

- Behaviour: If the dementia is related to kidney dialysis, the result is memory loss, loss of coordination and disorientation.

The most well known symptoms are:

- Alzheimer's
- Amyotrophic lateral sclerosis
- Anemia
- Colitis
- Hypothyroid
- Immune disorders
- Kidney dysfunction
- Liver dysfunction
- Neuromuscular disorders
- Parkinson's
- Ulcers

Where do we get the aluminum?

- Aluminum cans for beer, juice, and sodas
- Anti-perspirants
- Baking powder
- Bleached flour
- Drinking water
- Foods cooked in aluminum foil
- Medications, antacids
- Prepared foods made with tap water containing aluminum, salt containing aluminum
- Processed cheese
- Table salt

Arsenic – Used in pesticides and may be found in commercial wines, beers, fruits, vegetables, etc. It may be added in up to 70% of chicken feed (Roxsarone) and thus is found in both chickens and chicken eggs. Also found in pork feed and drinking water.

An interesting article on Arsenic and the USDA/FDA Cover up can be found on: http://drlwilson.com/articles/ARSENIC.htm

Symptoms include:

GUT:
- Abdominal pain
- Anorexia
- Diarrhea
- Enzyme inhibition
- Inhibits sulfhydryl enzymes, i.e. Glutathione transferase
- Interferes with folic acid (Vitamin B9) uptake
- Jaundice
- Kidney damage
- Liver dysfunction
- Stomatitis

OTHER:
- Abnormal ECG
- Edema
- Dermatitis
- Fever
- Fluid loss
- Goiter

- Hair loss
- Herpes
- Headache
- Impaired healing
- Sore throat
- Keratosis
- Muscle spasm
- Peripheral neuritis
- Stupor
- Vasodilation
- Vitiligo
- Weakness

It is also now recognized that arsenic toxicity:

- Alters signalling processes within cells
- Binds to thiols (Thiols are important in preventing free radicals and they act as cofactors for enzymes.)
- Causes oxidative stress
- Crosses the placenta and causes damage and still birth
- Triggers apoptosis (cell death)

Cadmium – Remember, zinc is required in over 100 critical enzymes and when depleted cadmium will step in. It is associated with aggression, violence and horror. Research indicates that high levels of cadmium in females tends to make them more male orientated, i.e. they act tough. Cadmium hardens various tissues and the arteries – making it difficult for the arteries to expand and contract. (Historically, this was only attributed to cholesterol).

Cadmium can be found in:
- Fish
- GMO foods
- Hydrogenated vegetable oils (margarine, peanut butter, shortening, etc.)
- Junk foods
- Plastic wraps for food
- Shellfish
- Strong coffees
- Water contamination

It is also associated with:

- Arthritis
- Birth defects
- Cancers of all kinds
- Degenerative diseases
- Developmental disorders
- Diabetes
- Heart disease
- Kidney disease
- Low sperm count
- Mental illness (ADHD, ADD, Autistic spectrum)

It is used in brake linings and consequently is widespread in the air.

Lead – Also associated with violent behaviour and ADHD, ADD, and lowered IQ and dementias. It can replace calcium in the bones, which can weaken them and cause osteoporosis. It can also replace calcium in the blood cells, which damages the blood cells and causes severe anemia. It can cross the blood brain barrier and replace vital brain minerals like magnesium and calcium.

It is also found on:
- Pesticides used on fruit, vegetables, and other foods
- Gasoline
- Lipstick
- Lubricants
- Medications
- Older house paints

It is associated with:

GUT:
- Abdominal pain
- Colic
- Constipation
- Liver dysfunction
- Weight loss

OTHER:
- Adrenal insufficiency
- Anemia
- Anxiety
- Arteriosclerosis
- Arthritis, osteo- and rheumatoid, and gout
- Brain function
- Concentration issues
- Convulsions
- Deafness

- Depression
- Dyslexia
- Encephalitis (acute inflammation of the brain)
- Epilepsy
- Fatigue
- Hallucinations
- Hypothyroidism
- Insomnia
- Low back pain
- Mood swings
- Multiple sclerosis
- Muscular dystrophy
- Schizophrenia
- Rickets
- Vertigo

Mercury – Mercury is recognized as the most toxic *and* the most common heavy metal. There are three different forms of mercury: methylmercury, elemental mercury (mercury vapours) and other mercury compounds. Inorganic mercury can cause damage to the gastrointestinal tract, the nervous system, and the kidneys and organic mercury is more readily absorbed through digestion. Mercury can attach to the hydrochloric acid in the stomach and produce mercuric chloride, which can damage the stomach lining and create ulcers.

Further down the gastrointestinal tract, mercury can destroy our much-needed friendly bacteria, not only allowing the overgrowth of candida (which can become systemic) but also having a massive compilation of other consequences. Deficiency or imbalances in the gut microbiota not only have a huge negative impact on the gut but also can have similar negative effects on almost all other systems in the body. In particular, they affect the two-way communications between the brain and gut, and between the liver and gut.[4]

Some claim that the organ most affected is the brain, which would be the result of methylmercury, which causes impaired neurological development and all kinds of cognitive issues. This is interesting in consideration that methylmercury is "readily and completely absorbed by the gastrointestinal tract". It attaches to cysteine (which we need for glutathione) and various proteins and peptides. When it attaches to transport proteins like methionine, it is not only carried throughout the body in the blood, but also crosses both the blood brain barrier and the placenta where it is absorbed by the fetus.[5]

Mercury also attaches to the hydrochloric acid in the stomach.

Mercury also has an affinity for fatty tissues; again this is mostly in the brain as the brain is about 70% fat. Consequently, it can have and enormous impact on the functioning of the brain.

Mercury activates an enzyme PLD (phospholipase D) that damages the cells lining the blood vessels, which provokes cholesterol (to patch up the damage) thus causing arteriosclerosis.

Mercury also displaces Vitamin C and consequently, one needs to have even more Vitamin C in their system.

It is often found along with copper toxicity and with other toxicities as well. It is often difficult to detect and simple blood or urine tests are virtually useless.

Methylmercury:

- Impairment in hearing
- Impairment in speech
- Impairment in walking
- Lack of coordination in movements
- Muscle weakness
- Peripheral vision impairment
- Pins and needles in extremities

Elemental mercury:

- Emotional issues
- Headaches
- Insomnia
- Irregular nerve responses
- Lowered cognitive performance

- Neuromuscular issues (weakness, atrophy, twitching)
- Tremors

Inorganic mercury:

- Memory loss
- Mental disturbances
- Mood swings
- Muscle weakness
- Skin rashes, i.e., dermatitis

Mercury poisoning in general has been associated with:

GUT:
- Acid reflux
- Allergies: due to damage of the gut wall and impairment of the gut flora
- Anorexia
- Bulimia
- Candida overgrowth (yeast infection)
- Colitis
- Constipation
- Crohn's disease
- Dysbiosis (imbalance in the microbiota which produce various types of waste by-products that cause discomfort in the gut)
- Flatulence (gas)
- Gastritis
- Hypoglycemia/hyperglycemia
- Irritable bowel syndrome

- Leaky gut syndrome
- Nausea and vomiting

OTHER:
- Acne – infections due to a suppressed immune system
- ADD (attention deficient disorder)
- ADHD (attention deficient hyperactivity disorder)
- Alzheimer's
- AML (amylotrophic lateral sclerosis)
- Aneurysm
- Anxiety and/or nervousness and/or panic attacks
- Apathy
- Arterial sclerosis
- Asthma
- Ataxia
- Autism
- Autoimmune diseases (methionine transport)
- Blood in the urine
- Borderline personality disorder
- Bruising
- Calcium elevated in the blood
- Cancer
- Cholesterol issues
- Circadian rhythm shifts (effects sleep cycle)
- Cognitive issues like memory, concentration, brain fog

- Dementias
- Depression and mood swings
- Dermatitis
- Dizziness
- Elevated homocysteine
- Fatigue
- Fibromyalgia
- Floaters (spots seen in front of the eyes)
- Grinding teeth while sleeping
- Headaches
- Hormonal issues
- Hypothyroidism
- Mineral deficiency, i.e., magnesium, selenium, zinc
- Muscle weakness and/or tremors
- Myasthemia gravis
- Obsessive compulsive disorders
- Parkinson's
- Rashes
- Sleep disorders
- Thyroid issues
- Tinnitus
- Vision – near-sighted and far-sighted, peripheral
- Vitamin deficiency, i.e., C
- Weight gain
- White coating on the tongue

Once again, it is important to note the domino effects that may be going on here. For instance, if mercury is absorbed by the hydrochloric acid in the stomach and then continues down the digestive tract to cause problems with the gut lining, this could lead to malabsorption of various nutrients and also allow for absorption of other damaging compounds. This also then impacts the gut bacteria, which is now recognized to have impact on various other parts of the body, i.e. the brain and the liver.

In addition, the mercury is now also being picked up by the blood, which is distributing it around the body, thus causing even more compound effects.

So where do we pick up all this mercury:

- Amalgams – old style fillings that not only have mercury but can also have numerous other toxicities
- Anti-fungal soaps, Ivory liquid, Dove soap,
- Bleaches
- Bleached flour
- Contact lens solutions
- Cosmetics
- Exhaust fumes
- Fabric softener
- Fish – coastal or in contaminated streams and lakes

- Medications: prescription, i.e. diuretics for blood pressure, antifungals, over-the-counter-drugs, vaccinations, all of which may contain thimerosal, which is a mercury compound used as a preservative
- Paints
- Shellfish

For a complete list go to:
www.drlwilson.com/articles/MERCURY.htm

Nickel – A particularly toxic metal that can also cause depression and suicidal thinking. It tends to accumulate in the kidneys but affects the lungs and the skin.

The symptoms from nickel toxicity include:

- Cancer (oral, intestinal and lung)
- Heart attacks
- Haemorrhaging
- Kidney dysfunction
- Low blood pressure
- Nausea and/or vomiting
- Skin issues

But we started out looking at heavy metal toxicity and the gut. So what specifically do we need to address?

- Leaky gut syndrome – penetration through the gut lining allowing both nutrients and toxins to flow into areas they should not be.
- Harm to the gut bacteria – required for so many different functions in the body and in particular they support our immune system. But the wrong type of gut bacteria can cause problems from obesity and diabetes to depression, Parkinson's, Alheimer's, schizophrenia, high blood pressure, liver issues and a number of other issues.[6,7]

NINE

Microbes, Inflammation, and the Gut

We have a massive quantity of good bacteria in our gut—or at least we should have. In a healthy body there are more good bacteria in the gut than cells in the entire body!

There are therefore, more of them than there is of us. How do you incorporate that into your perception of self-identity? Okay, we won't go there right now.

There have been a great number of studies on our gut's bacteria, a.k.a. microbiota in the last couple of years. These microbes can provide an enormous benefit, and if they are in the wrong ratios or are depleted they can do enormous harm.

In fact, there is a growing consensus among biologists that we should not separate an organism's genetic load from the context of its microbiota! What does that mean?

Well, we used to think that the brains of the cells were in the genetic code. Then we realized that the genes were simply the reproductive center of the cell.

But now, we are looking at whether the microbiota in the system can alter the genes!

What are the research studies revealing in humans?

- When they profile the microbiota of twins who are obese and lean, they find that there are major differences:
  - When the whole environment is analyzed, i.e. the bacteria and enzymes, which then results in the manner that the carbohydrates, lipids, and amino acids are metabolized, the profile is significantly different between those who are obese versus those who are lean.
- Type I diabetes – conventional medicine assumes that both Type I and Type II diabetes are non-reversible.
  - Alternative medicine has shown that Type II is easily reversible but has a more difficult process with Type I.
  - Type I diabetes can lead to or co-occur with:
    - Aberrant intestinal microbiota
    - Leaky intestinal mucosal barrier
    - Intrinsic differences in immune responsiveness

When compared to healthy children, autoimmune children revealed:

- Unstable gut biomes
- Decreased levels of species diversity
- Unhealthy Firmicutes replace healthy bacteriodetes

We now know that the microbiota have an impact on the immune system (most of which is in the gut). Consequently, our understanding of the immune system is changing. The "old view" identifies the immune system as a complex organization of molecules, cells, tissues, and organs that work in synchrony to fight the pathogens – the predominant factor in the old "Germ Theory".

However, now we have to accept that perhaps there might be as much control by the microbes on the immune system, as there is control of the immune system on the microbes.

For instance, it is now recognized that some microbiota affect Th17 cell differentiation in the gut mucosa, which are known to play a role in inflammatory processes and the following disorders:

- Autoimmune uveitis
- Crohn's disease
- Juvenile diabetes
- Multiple sclerosis
- Psoriasis
- Rheumatoid arthritis[1,2]

In fact, researchers are now looking at classifying people in accordance with their gut microbiota. Research is now suggesting that there are perhaps three major categories that respond differently to diet and drug intake. [3]

Perhaps when dealing with the various inflammatory disorders, we need to start looking at how to enhance various gut microbiota.

The microbiota don't just reside in the gut; they reside throughout the body. For instance, we all know that the skin is the largest organ. There are numerous different profiles of microbiota in different areas of the skin, i.e. the hair, the feet, under the arms, etc. Even skin microbes that dwell in close proximity can have significant differences, i.e. between those found on the neck and the underarm.

These microbes protect against pathogens entering the body through the skin. They also contribute to the regulation of moisture loss, body temperature and other functions. In fact, they represent an entirely different type of ecosystem in the human body.

Studies are now expanding from the understanding of the gut bacteria to the bacterial profiles found in different areas of the skin and the link between skin, microbiota and health/disease and we will probably find connection with inflammatory markers here, too.[4]

TEN

Correlations Between Gut Inflammatory Disorders and Other Disorders

The gut, whether we look at toxins, microbiota, or any other variable, is connected to the rest of the body. Conventional medicine took a long time to recognize this while alternative medicine has always embraced this knowledge.

The more historical connection between the gut and other disorders focused on issues resulting from:

1. Food and thus nutrients get metabolized in the gut – therefore, the gut was, in effect, the source of nutrients required by the body.

2. Toxicity in the gut results in inflammation in the gut and can thus have an impact on what is absorbed versus what is eliminated.

In recent research we have to expand this idea to include that:

1. The mind can have a huge impact on the gut and how it functions.
2. The microbiota in the gut can impact:
   a. what is digested
   b. what is absorbed
   c. what is eliminated
   d. what leaks through the gut mucosa.

We have looked at how *and* now we have to include even more variables:

1. There is a two-way connection between the gut and the brain.
2. The microbe in the gut can impact the rest of the body through:
   e. The vagus nerve – to the brain
   f. Through the immune system –
      i. T cells, i.e., Th17
      ii. Tumour necrosis cells
      iii. Natural killer cells.

Let's look at some specific issues that have an impact:

1) **Constipation and Depression**
   a. This may be the result of the medication itself, i.e. the drugs cause the constipation. A quick look at what is going on here reveals that low serotonin has never been shown to be the cause of depression nor has regulating it ever been shown to eliminate depression. Furthermore, the gut makes over 90% of the body's serotonin. So when a depressed client is prescribed serotonin – what is it doing to the serotonin produced in the gut?
   b. Depression is also linked with a general "slowing" down of the body's systems and this may include the gut

system, which is stimulated by the 10th cranial nerve, the vagus nerve.

  c. Constipation may be caused from lack of nutrients, which then also affects the brain, i.e. magnesium, various B vitamins.

  d. Constipation may be the result of toxicities, which may also impact the absorption of nutrients and elimination of toxins but also inflammatory issues.[1]

2) **The gut, the immune system and Multiple Sclerosis**

  a. The gut bacteria communicate with the immune cells by secreting various molecules, which communicate back by releasing various molecules and compounds.

  b. These various compounds can provoke, inhibit, or regulate various other compounds that allow for MS to develop or inhibit the process.[2]

3) **Autism, Digestion and Inflammation**

  a. The inflammatory system is part of the immune system, and the majority of the immune system is in the gut. Thus the gut is the primary regulator of the inflammatory system.

  b. The innate immune system plays a role in the defence against microbes.

c. Children with autism have a higher rate of inflammation and immune system dysregulation in the digestive tract than children without the disorder.
d. Causes of inflammatory disorders, in children, in the gut include:
    i.   Toxicity
    ii. Heavy metal toxicity
    iii. Lack of transfer factor due to insufficient mother's milk
    iv. Vaccinations.

ELEVEN

Anti-Inflammatory Diet

As you can see, there are lots of reasons for inflammation and there are lots of problems because of inflammation.

As noted earlier, inflammation is the cause of most diseases and dysfunctions in today's world of chronic illnesses and disorders.

The most effective health practitioner is the one who is going to get to the root cause of the problem. The more specific one can be about the root source, the more specified the treatment protocol can be.

Unfortunately, diagnosis is not within the capability of this book so I cannot provide any specific treatments. What the book can do is provide a simplified protocol for inflammation in general.

We will look at some different components here:
- Tips for an anti-inflammatory diet
- Anti-inflammatory foods
- Inflammatory foods
- Some meal examples
- Beneficial supplements
- Essential oils

First, let's look at some anti-inflammatory and inflammatory foods, beginning with anti-inflammatory foods:

Category	Benefit	Food
Fish	Omega 3s – anti-inflammatory EPAs and DHAs fatty acids	Fatty Fish: salmon, mackerel, tuna, sardines, anchovies
Other sea products	Fucoidan (anti-inflammatory, anti-tumor and anti-oxidant	Kelp
Plants: Vegetables	Cytokines, Sulfuraphane, Vit. E, Calcium, Iron	Dark Leafy greens: broccoli, collard greens, kale, spinach,
	Lycopene	Nightshade Vegetables: Peppers and Tomatoes
	Betalaines, Vit. C, fiber	Beets
	Vit. A, beta-carotene, magnesium, manganese, Vit. B2, B6, B9, C, E, K, calcium, iron	Roots: carrots, squash, sweet potatoes
	Beta-cryptoxanthin	Pumpkin
Plants: Fruit		Apples, blueberries,

		cherries, pineapple, raspberries,
	Vit C and E, bromelain – as effective as NSAIDs	Pineapple, papaya
	Anti-oxidants, anti-inflammatories, magnesium	Chocolate – 100%
Mushrooms	Polysaccrides: Beta-glycans immune boosters	Shiitake, Maitake, Cordyceps, Enoki, Oyster
Spices	Quercetin and allicin	Garlic and onions
Spices	Curcumin turns off NF Kappa B inflammatory	Turmeric, ginger, especially good for Crohn's
Spice	When minerals are taken together they are more effective	Mineral salt or Sea salt
Spices		Basil, chili peppers, oregano, rosemary, thyme
Seeds	Omega 3s, fibre, minerals	Chia/Salba, Hemp, Ground Flax, Sunflower, Pumpkin, Sesame, Amaranth

Nuts	Omega 3s – anti-inflammatory fatty acids and fibre, calcium, and Vit. E	Almonds, Walnuts, Hazelnuts, Pecans, Brazil nuts
Fermented foods	Pre- and Probiotics	Sauerkraut, Pickled beets, Asparagus, Yogurt, Kefir,
Fibres	Reduce levels of C-reactive proteins, Vit. E	Whole grains, German rye, Sourdough, Sprouted Grains
Teas	ECGCs and anti-oxidants	Green tea, Rooibos, ginger, bergamot – Earl Grey
Dairy	Vitamin D	Yogurt
Oils	Omega 3s	Almond, Sesame, Avocado, Grape seed

And then we have the inflammatory foods:

Category	Food
Meats	Processed, smoked, deli, packaged foods, feedlot raised meats
Plants: Vegetables	Potatoes, white rice, French fries, onion rings, potato chips, nachos
Plants: Fruit	Strawberries: have a high affinity for mercury
	Unless 100% Chocolate – detrimental

Sugars	High fructose corn syrups, dextrose, fructose, syrups, maltose, sorghum syrup sucrose, artificial/synthetic sugars: Aspartame, NutraSweet, Splenda, etc.
Artificial food additives	MSG (Monosodium Glutamate), Aspartame
Processed foods	Soups, microwaved, pasteurized
Spices	Iodized table salt
Food additives	Colors, flavour enhances, stabilizers, preservatives: Sulphites, benzoates, etc.
Nuts	Peanuts – actually legumes have high probability of Aspergillus fungus.
Fermented foods	Store bought fermented foods do not have the quality of probiotics that homemade do.
Fibres	White and brown breads, whole wheat bread, multigrain breads, baking goods, deserts
Teas	Teas full of sugars and artificial flavourings
Coffee	Highly toxic
Alcohol	High in sugar and a burden to the liver
Other drinks	Sodas, energy drinks,
Dairy	Pasteurized foods have eliminated the good food nutrients: Ice cream, milk, processed cheeses

Oils	Most olive oil is full of cheaper oils and artificial omega 3s; margarine, shortening, lard

If we put together an anti-inflammatory pyramid, it would look like this:

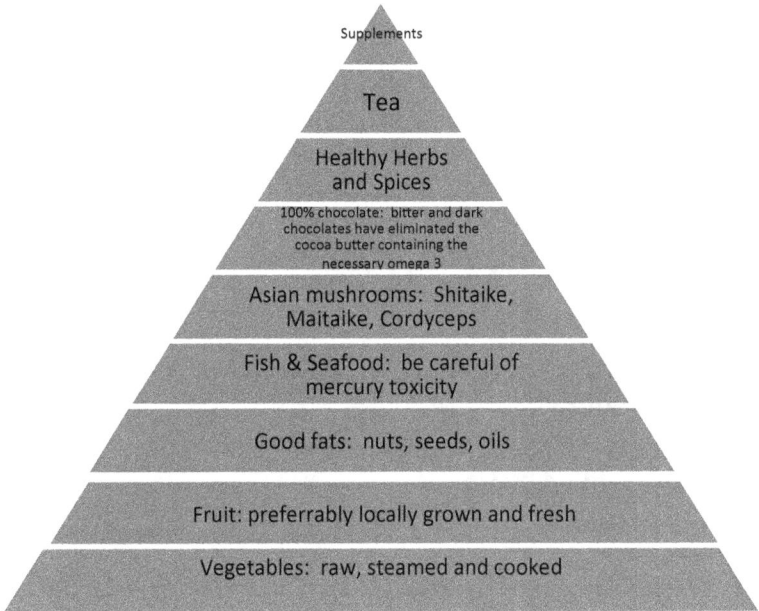

Supplements

Tea

Healthy Herbs and Spices

100% chocolate: bitter and dark chocolates have eliminated the cocoa butter containing the necessary omega 3

Asian mushrooms: Shitaike, Maitaike, Cordyceps

Fish & Seafood: be careful of mercury toxicity

Good fats: nuts, seeds, oils

Fruit: preferrably locally grown and fresh

Vegetables: raw, steamed and cooked

We can also suggest Essential oils that are known for their anti-inflammatory capacity:

- Thyme
- Rose
- Clove
- Eucalyptus
- Bergamot
- Fennel
- Copaiba [1]

Supplements:

- Fish oil
- Krill
- Omega 3s
- Flax seed oil
- Anti-oxidants
- Alpha Lipoic Acid
- Bioflavonoids
- Black willow
- Borage or Star Flower Oil
- Boswellia
- Bromelain
- CoQ10
- Curcumin
- Ginger
- Licorice
- Milk Thistle
- Resveratrol
- Vitamin C, E,
- Zinc

The following is a good anti-inflammatory menu:

DAY 1

Breakfast:
Steel cut oats with cinnamon, cardamom, nutmeg, cloves and blueberries
Top with coconut or almond milk

Lunch:
Pumpkin soup with ginger:

3 cans pumpkin
5 C chicken broth
2 C milk
½ C heavy cream
¼ C coconut sugar
2 chopped medium yellow onions
2 Tsp. minced garlic
Crushed red pepper
Curry powder
Cayenne pepper

Sauté onions in butter; add spices.
Add pumpkin, chicken broth, blend and bring to a boil. Reduce heat for about 10 minutes. Transfer soup to blender and blend in batches till smooth. Transfer back to pot on low heat and while stirring, add coconut sugar, then milk, followed by the cream. Add remaining spices and stir. Heat until warm and serve.

Beet and Spinach salad:
  4 cooked and sliced beets
  4 C packed fresh spinach
  1 chopped green apple
  2 green onions
Dressing: Apple cider vinegar, avocado oil, Dijon mustard, salt, pepper, garlic.

Dinner:
Turmeric stir-fry with organic chicken
  Organic chicken
  Red and green onions
  Asian mushrooms
  Broccoli

Red/green/yellow/orange peppers (if you don't have a reaction to nightshade vegetables)

DAY 2

Breakfast:
Omelette made with:
      2 free range
      Onions
      Mushrooms
      Red/orange/yellow/green peppers
      Top with Asiago cheese

Lunch:
Coleslaw:
      Red and green cabbage
      Shredded carrots
      Chopped red and white onions
      Broccoli
      Cauliflower
      Sesame and sliced almonds
      Pineapple
      Dried cranberries
      Shredded lime and orange peel
Dressing: Mayonnaise and apple cider vinegar

Dinner:
Broiled salmon with mayonnaise and dill
Boiled kale with peanut sauce
Greek salad:
      Tomato
      Cucumber
      Green pepper

Red onions
Sliced avocado
Sliced olives
Feta cheese
Dressing: Avocado oil and balsamic vinegar,
oregano, salt and pepper.

DAY 3

Breakfast:
Greek yogurt with greens powder

Lunch:
Kippers or smoked herring on a salad:
      Romaine lettuce
      Cucumber
      Red and green peppers
      Red and green onions
      Mushrooms
      Tomatoes
Slice of sourdough bread (homemade much better)

Dinner:
Bowl of chili with sour cream

DAY 4

Breakfast:
Homemade granola with almond or coconut milk:

(We know that all the above are good for you, so
let's put them into a homemade recipe. This is my
own granola recipe.)

Coconut Honey Almond Granola

Ingredients:

- 1 C almonds – I prefer mine slivered
- 3 C oats – the old fashioned kind, not some quick mix that is devoid of nutrient
- ½ C coconut flakes
- ½ tsp mineral salt
- 1/3 brown sugar, jiggery sugar, beet sugar – any sugar that is not processed – or if you would prefer use 1 Tbsp stevia
- 1/3 C honey – unprocessed – but other than that you choose the kind, alfalfa, blueberry, burdock, etc
- 3 Tbsp coconut oil
- ¼ tsp vanilla extract
- 1/8 tsp almond extract

Directions:

1. Pour almonds, oats, salt, sugar into a bowl and mix
2. Heat honey and oil in a small saucepan; then add vanilla and almond extracts
3. Pour honey mix over oat mix
4. Lay out mixture on a parchment – bake at 350F for 5 min
5. Stir and bake for another 5 min
6. Allow to cool, break apart, store in a glass jar with a tight lid

Lunch:
Coleslaw – as above
Dinner:
Spinach salad:
 ½ lb. spinach torn into small pieces
 ¾ C silvered almonds
 1 C dried cranberries
 2 Tbsp. sesame seeds
 2 Tsp. minced onion
Dressing:
 ¼ C Apple cider vinegar
 ¼ C wine vinegar
 ¼ Tsp. paprika
 ½ C sesame oil

Sweet potato
Broiled tilapia with mayonnaise and dill

DAY 5

Breakfast:
2 poached eggs
Sourdough bread

Lunch:
Coleslaw – as above

Dinner:
Broccoli and cauliflower salad
 5 C broccoli – chopped into small pieces
 5 C cauliflower – chopped into small pieces
 2/3 C chopped onions (red, white, green)
 2 C shredded cheddar cheese
 ¼ C sunflower and sesame seeds

1/3 C raisins
Dressing:
    1 C mayonnaise
    1 Tbsp. apple cider vinegar
    1 Tbsp. red wine
Sweet potato and sour cream
Broiled tilapia with mayonnaise and dill

DAY 6

Breakfast:
Greek yogurt with greens powder

Lunch:
Coleslaw as above

Dinner:
Spinach salad as above
Sweet potato
Broiled tilapia with mayonnaise and dill

DAY 7

Breakfast:
2 blueberry crepes:
    ¾ C gluten free flour baking mix
    6 C blueberries
    2 Tbsp. honey
    4 large eggs
    1 C almond milk
    2 Tbsp sesame oil
    1 Tsp. vanilla extract
       1 Tablespoon coconut sugar
       Dash of mineral salt

Mix blueberries and coconut sugar and set aside. Whisk together gluten free mix, honey, sugar, and salt. Whisk together eggs, milk, and vanilla. Whisk dry ingredients into wet ingredients. Pour onto hot skillet. Cook till brown and flip for about 10 seconds.

Lunch:
Beet salad:
    2 bunches cooked beets
    1 Onion
    Walnuts
    Argula
    Goat cheese
Dressing: Sesame oil, red wine vinegar/apple cider vinegar, mineral salt, pepper
Alternate Dressing: Sesame oil, apple cider vinegar, chopped fresh mint, Dijon mustard, mineral salt, pepper

Dinner:
Sauerkraut
Black Bean Burgers
    ½ C mayonnaise
    1 lime
    ½ Tsp. hot sauce
    1 minced jalapeno
    2 minced garlic cloves
    1 chopped onion
    2 cans black beans (drained and rinsed)
    2 C grated raw sweet potato
    1 C plain breadcrumbs
    1 Sourdough bun

Squeeze lime into bowl, add mayonnaise and hot sauce, stir and refrigerate. Gently fry onions, jalapeno, garlic and turmeric and put into a bowl. Add in mashed black beans, sweet potato, egg and ½ the breadcrumbs and stir. Create about 8 patties and place on a cookie sheet. Broil 8 – 10 minutes per side. Serve with lime mayonnaise.

Appendix 1

Hippocrates:

A wise man should consider that health is the greatest of human blessings, and learn how by his own thought to derive benefit from his illness.

It is more important to know what sort of a person has a disease than to know what sort of disease a person has. (This is why all practitioners should also be psychologists.)

Natural forces within us are the true healers of disease. (This is why no practitioner should ever be arrogant about his or her abilities.)

Whenever a doctor cannot do good, he or she must be kept from doing harm. (The problem is that so many are taught harmful ways of managing symptoms.)

Wherever the art of medicine is loved, there is also a love of humanity. (Unfortunately, the love might be intricately tied in with greed and/or ego.)

Extreme remedies are very appropriate for extreme diseases.

To do nothing is also a good remedy (allow the body to do what was designed to do).

A physician without knowledge of astrology has no right to call himself or herself a physician (I love this one.) Ayurvedic medicine has a whole branch in Ayurvedic Astrology, which has been shown to have a strong correlation with what goes on in the body.

Everything in excess is opposed to nature.

Quotes:

Chapter 6

[1] Shing, CM, et al. Nutritional compounds influence tissue factor expression and inflammation of chronic kidney disease in patients in vitro. Found in: ncbi.nlm.nih.gov/pubmed/21295946

Chapter 7

[1] Conterno, Lorenza, et al. Obesity and the gut microbiota: does up-regulating colonic fermentation protect against obesity and metabolic disease? Found in: http://www.ncbi.nlm.nih.gov/pmc/articles/PMC3145060/

Chapter 8

[1] Stellpflug, Craig. Myth Busted: Vaccinations are not Immunizations. Found in: http://www.infowars.com/myth-busted-vaccinations-are-not-immunizations/

[2] Synergistic Effects of Mercury with Other Toxic Metals: Extreme Synergistic Toxicity. Found in: http://www.flcv.com/hgsynerg.html

[3] International Programme on Chemical Safety. Found in: http://www.who.int/ipcs/assessment/public_health/chemicals_phc/en/

[4] Methylmercury. Found in:
http://en.wikipedia.org/wiki/Methylmercury

[5] Methylmercury. Found in:
http://en.wikipedia.org/wiki/Methylmercury

[6] Metabolic Healing. Found in:
http://metabolichealing.com/gut-function-intestinal-mucosal-barrier/

[7] Step II Easy Step Detoxification Personal Guide.
Found in:
http://cyhvids.s3.amazonaws.com/Step%202%20Detox%20Capture%20Your%20Health%202.pdf

Chapter 9

[1] Cha, Aye-Ran, et al. Downregulation of TH17 cells in the Small Intestine by Disruption of Gut Flora in the Absence of Retinoic Acid. Found in:
http://www.jimmunol.org/content/184/12/6799.full

[2] Microbiome. Found in:
http://en.wikipedia.org/wiki/Microbiome

[3] Enterotypes of the human gut microbiome. Found in:
http://www-huber.embl.de/pub/pdf/Arumugam_Nature_2011.pdf

[4] Structure, function and diversity of the healthy human microbiome. Found in:

http://www.nature.com/nature/journal/v486/n74 02/full/nature11234.html

Chapter 10

[1] Daniels, Jennifer. Depression via Constipation. Found in:
http://www.rense.com/general66/depress.htm

[2] King, Mary. A gut reaction to MS: Exploring possible links between the gut, the immune system and MS. Found in:
http://www.momentummagazineonline.com/gut-reaction-ms/

Chapter 11

[1] 6 Proven Anti-Inflammatory Essential oils You Should Be Using. Found in:
http://theconsciouslife.com/6-natural-anti-inflammatory-essential-oils.htm

References:

http://www.ncbi.nlm.nih.gov/pubmed/10858024

http://www.ncbi.nlm.nih.gov/pubmed/12617463

http://pubs.acs.org/doi/abs/10.1021/bk-2001-0788.ch007

http://en.wikipedia.org/wiki/Docosahexaenoic_acid

http://www.emergencybocadentist.com/news/xocxai_Mega.pdf

http://www.livestrong.com/article/522058-foods-containing-cis-fats/

http://ebm.rsmjournals.com/content/229/3/215.full

Mercury poisoning. Found on:
http://www.medicinenet.com/mercury_poisoning/page3.htm#what_are_the_health_effects_and_symptoms_of_mercury_exposure_or_poisoning

http://drlwilson.com/articles/MERCURY.htm

http://www.lef.org/protocols/prtcls-txt/t-prtcl-156.htm

http://www.lenntech.com/processes/heavy/heavy-metals/heavy-metals.htm

www.ingramcontent.com/pod-product-compliance
Lightning Source LLC
Chambersburg PA
CBHW030315220326
41519CB00069B/6105